Con

Chapter

Chapter 1

Hypnotherapy Expertise: 30 Years with Dr David Postlethwaite

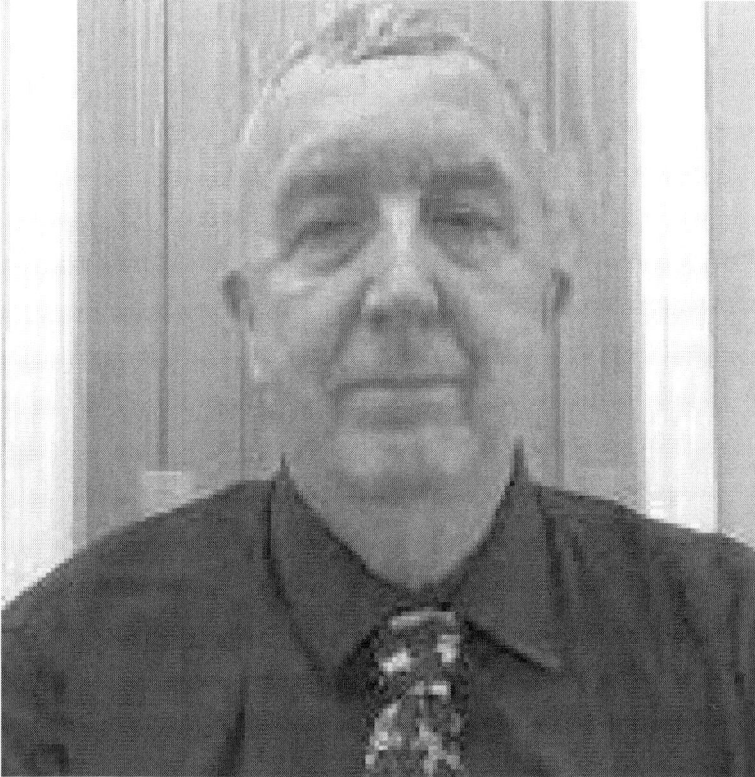

Hypnotherapy is a powerful tool that has been used for centuries to help individuals overcome a variety of challenges, from phobias to addictions. One expert in the field who has been making a significant impact for over three decades is Dr David Postlethwaite. With a wealth of experience and a unique approach to hypnotherapy, Dr David has helped countless clients achieve transformative results in just one session. In this chapter, we will delve into Dr David's expertise, his innovative one session model, the science behind hypnotherapy, success stories from his clients, his global influence and recognition, the importance of the therapeutic relationship, future directions in hypnotherapy, and how to access his sessions.

A Journey Through Three Decades

Embarking on a professional path that would ultimately redefine the contours of hypnotherapy, Dr David Postlethwaite embarked upon his remarkable career over thirty years ago. This span, stretching across three rich decades, has been characterised by a profound commitment to evolving and perfecting the art of hypnotherapy. Not content with resting on the laurels of established methodologies, Dr David has consistently sought to push the boundaries of what is possible within the realm of therapeutic intervention. His journey, illuminated by a curious and innovative spirit, has taken him across the globe, allowing him to amass a treasure trove of cultural insights and experiences that have significantly informed his practice.

In the early stages of his career, Dr David recognised the transformative potential of hypnotherapy. He observed its power not just in treating superficial symptoms, but in addressing the deep-seated emotional and psychological foundations of various issues. This insight propelled him to delve deeper into the science and technique of hypnotherapy, grounding his approach in the rich interplay between mind, body, and emotional well-being. His pursuit of knowledge was not confined to the shores of his home country. Instead, Dr David sought to globalise his understanding of human psychology, working with clients from diverse cultural backgrounds. This exposure to a wide range of human experiences has been pivotal in shaping his holistic approach to hypnotherapy.

Throughout the years, Dr David has been a keen observer of the evolving landscape of mental health and therapeutic practices. He has witnessed first-hand the shifts in societal attitudes towards mental health, from scepticism and misunderstanding to a growing acceptance and appreciation of the importance of mental well-being. This changing tide has provided both challenges and opportunities, inspiring Dr David to continuously refine his approach to meet the needs of his clients in a rapidly evolving world.

His travels and work abroad have not only enriched his personal and professional life but have also allowed him to leave a lasting impact on the hypnotherapy field worldwide. Dr David has been instrumental in introducing his pioneering one session model to different corners of the globe, demonstrating its efficacy and efficiency in bringing about significant psychological change. This model, grounded in his extensive experience and deep understanding of human psychology, has challenged traditional practices and set new benchmarks for success in the field of hypnotherapy.

As Dr David navigated through these three decades, his journey has been more than just a personal or professional quest. It has been a journey of discovery, learning, and above all, healing.

The One Session Model Explained

The one session model, pioneered by Dr David Postlethwaite, represents a significant departure from conventional hypnotherapy practices. Traditionally, hypnotherapy has been perceived as a lengthy process, often requiring numerous sessions to effect any real change. Dr David, drawing on his extensive experience and profound understanding of the human psyche, has innovatively condensed this process into a single, powerful session. This approach not only challenges traditional methods but redefines the potential for rapid and effective therapeutic transformation.

At the core of the one session model is a meticulously structured process that leverages an intense, focused approach to hypnotherapy. Dr David harnesses the full spectrum of his expertise to engage with the client's subconscious mind deeply and efficiently. The session is designed to unearth and address the root causes of the client's issue, rather than merely managing symptoms. This depth of engagement with the subconscious ensures that the changes are not just immediate but also enduring.

The model is underpinned by a bespoke treatment plan tailored to the unique needs and circumstances of each client. Prior to the session, Dr David conducts a thorough assessment to understand the client's history, challenges, and objectives. This preparatory work is crucial in crafting a session that is both highly personalised and targeted, maximising the potential for a successful outcome.

A crucial element of the one session model's success lies in its empowering nature. Clients are not just passive recipients of therapy; they are active participants in their journey towards healing. Dr David equips them with the tools and strategies needed to sustain their newfound well-being beyond the session. This empowerment aspect ensures that the benefits of the one session model extend far into the future, embedding positive changes within the client's life.

The efficacy of this model is a testament to Dr David's skill and the sophisticated understanding of hypnotherapy's potential. By condensing the therapeutic process into a single, impactful session, he has not only broadened access to hypnotherapy but has also illuminated the path towards a more efficient and effective form of psychological intervention. This model stands as a beacon for those seeking profound change within a limited timeframe, reflecting Dr David's commitment to innovation and excellence in the field of hypnotherapy.

The Science Behind Hypnotherapy

Hypnotherapy, a modality rooted in the intricate workings of the subconscious mind, operates on the principle that our deepest beliefs and patterns lie beneath our conscious awareness. Dr David Postlethwaite, leveraging decades of clinical experience and an astute understanding of cognitive processes, applies this therapeutic technique to initiate profound and lasting change within individuals. The efficacy of hypnotherapy is grounded in its ability to directly communicate with the subconscious, bypassing the critical faculties of the conscious mind to instigate behavioural, emotional, and psychological transformations.

Central to the success of hypnotherapy is the state of hypnosis, a naturally occurring, trance-like condition in which individuals are more open to suggestions and changes in perception. During this state, the focused attention of the client allows for a heightened receptivity to therapeutic interventions. Dr David skilfully induces this state, employing a combination of relaxation techniques and guided imagery to facilitate a deep internal focus. It is within this state that the subconscious can be effectively reprogrammed to alter unwanted behaviours and patterns, laying the groundwork for lasting change.

Neuroscientific research underpins the mechanisms of hypnotherapy, illuminating how brainwave patterns alter during hypnosis. These alterations suggest a shift towards a more receptive and malleable state, enabling the therapeutic suggestions made by Dr David to be more deeply embedded within the subconscious. Furthermore, advances in neuroimaging have provided insights into how hypnosis can modulate activity in specific areas of the brain associated with attention, suggestion, and pain perception, offering a biological basis for its efficacy.

Hypnotherapy's versatility is reflected in its application across a multitude of psychological and behavioural issues. Through tailored hypnotic suggestions, Dr David addresses the underlying causes of these issues, from phobias and anxiety to addictive behaviours and self-esteem challenges. The science behind hypnotherapy supports its use as a holistic tool, not merely alleviating symptoms but fostering an environment for the root of the issue to be confronted and resolved.

The therapeutic potential of hypnotherapy, championed by Dr David Postlethwaite, is bolstered by a growing body of empirical evidence. Randomised controlled trials and meta-analyses have corroborated the effectiveness of hypnotherapy in improving mental health outcomes, underscoring its legitimacy and value as a therapeutic modality. This scientific framework, combined with Dr David's innovative one session model, amplifies the transformative capacity of hypnotherapy, offering a potent, science-backed avenue for personal change and healing.

Transformative Success Stories
The remarkable efficacy of Dr David Postlethwaite's hypnotherapy sessions is best exemplified through the life-altering experiences of his clients. Over the years, numerous individuals have turned to Dr David seeking relief from a myriad of psychological and behavioural challenges. Each success story stands as a powerful testament to the transformative potential of hypnotherapy, particularly the pioneering one session model developed by Dr David.

One striking narrative involves a client who had been grappling with severe claustrophobia for decades. This debilitating fear had restricted her ability to travel, pursue certain careers, and even partake in routine activities. Skeptical yet desperate for a solution, she underwent a session with Dr David. To her astonishment, she found herself boarding a flight without the paralysing anxiety that had shadowed her for years, just days after the session. This profound change opened new avenues in her life, allowing her to explore opportunities previously marred by fear.

Another narrative centres on an individual battling a smoking addiction that had persisted unchecked for over twenty years. Traditional cessation methods had failed, leaving him in a cycle of guilt and relapse. After a single hypnotherapy session with Dr David, he discovered an unprecedented sense of control. Weeks turned into months, and he remained smoke-free. This transformative experience not only improved his physical health but also instilled a newfound confidence in his ability to conquer other long-standing habits.

Further testimonials reveal the scope of Dr David's expertise, spanning cases of severe anxiety, insomnia, and even chronic pain management. Clients who had resigned themselves to a life dominated by their conditions found relief and empowerment in just one session. The feedback consistently highlights not just the immediate impact of the therapy, but its durability—clients report sustained improvements, a testament to the depth at which the hypnotherapy works.

These stories underscore the unique and profound impact of Dr David's one session model. It is not merely the breadth of issues addressed but the depth of change achieved that sets his practice apart. Each client's journey from distress to wellness adds to the compelling narrative of Dr David Postlethwaite's contributions to the field of hypnotherapy, reinforcing the potential for genuine, lasting transformation through his specialised approach.

Global Influence and Recognition

The global footprint of Dr David Postlethwaite in the sphere of hypnotherapy is both extensive and profound. His pioneering work, particularly the one session model, has traversed national boundaries, bringing about a paradigm shift in the therapeutic practices across continents. Dr David's professional odyssey has seen him sharing his knowledge and expertise in numerous countries, where his methods have been embraced with enthusiasm by both practitioners and clients alike.

This worldwide recognition is not merely a testament to the effectiveness of his unique approach but also speaks volumes about the universal applicability of his techniques. Dr David's ability to adapt his methods to suit diverse cultural contexts has been pivotal in broadening the appeal and acceptance of hypnotherapy on a global scale. His travels and professional engagements across different cultures have enriched his practice, imbuing it with a depth of understanding and sensitivity towards the nuances of varied human experiences and psychological needs.

In every country he has worked, Dr David has left an indelible mark on both the professional community and those he has helped. His workshops and seminars are highly sought after, drawing attendees from far and wide who are keen to learn from his insights and adopt his innovative methods. The accolades and recognition that have come his way are a reflection of the impact he has had on the global hypnotherapy landscape.
Moreover, Dr David's contributions to international conferences and symposiums on hypnotherapy and mental health have further cemented his status as an authority in the field. Through these platforms, he has not only disseminated his findings and methodologies but has also engaged in valuable exchanges with fellow professionals, contributing to the ongoing evolution of hypnotherapy as a respected and effective therapeutic modality.

His global influence extends into the digital realm as well, where his online sessions have made his expertise accessible to clients worldwide, breaking geographical barriers and bringing about transformational change in the lives of individuals across the globe. Through these varied channels, Dr David Postlethwaite continues to shape the practice of hypnotherapy, ensuring its growth and relevance in addressing the psychological and emotional well-being of people everywhere.

The Therapeutic Relationship

At the heart of Dr David Postlethwaite's hypnotherapy practice lies the pivotal role of the therapeutic relationship. This bond between therapist and client is not merely ancillary; it is foundational to the process and success of the therapy. Dr David's mastery in fostering this relationship stems from his deep understanding that the efficacy of hypnotherapy is intrinsically linked to the quality of connection established. He approaches each interaction with empathy, respect, and an openness that encourages clients to reciprocate in kind, creating a milieu of mutual trust and safety.

In the realm of hypnotherapy, where clients are guided to explore and confront their vulnerabilities and subconscious barriers, the significance of a secure therapeutic relationship cannot be overstated. Dr David's skill in building this rapport is evident in his ability to make clients feel understood, valued, and empowered. He listens intently, validates their experiences, and tailors his therapeutic approach to reflect their individual needs and personalities. This personalised engagement is crucial, as it not only enhances the client's comfort and readiness to engage in the hypnotherapeutic process but also optimises the receptiveness of their subconscious to therapeutic suggestions.

Dr David recognises that the journey through hypnotherapy is a shared endeavour; a collaborative exploration where therapist and client are partners in pursuit of healing and transformation. This collaborative spirit is a hallmark of his sessions, inviting clients to play an active role in their journey towards well-being. By demystifying the process of hypnotherapy and involving clients in crafting their therapeutic goals, Dr David ensures that the journey is empowering and aligned with the client's aspirations.

Moreover, the strength of the therapeutic relationship extends beyond the confines of the session itself. It is the cornerstone upon which the resilience and continuity of the therapeutic outcomes rest. Dr David's commitment to this relationship underscores his dedication not just to the immediate success of the therapy but to the long-term well-being of his clients. In essence, the therapeutic relationship cultivated by Dr David Postlethwaite is a profound alliance, one that nurtures trust, fosters growth, and facilitates enduring change, embodying the very essence of effective hypnotherapy.

Future Directions in Hypnotherapy
In the ever-evolving landscape of mental health and therapeutic practices, hypnotherapy stands on the brink of transformative advancements. Dr David Postlethwaite, with his pioneering one session model and decades of invaluable insight, is poised to propel the field into new realms of efficacy and accessibility. As we look towards the horizon, several areas emerge as pivotal to the future trajectory of hypnotherapy, guided by Dr David's innovative spirit.

Technological Integration and Digital Therapeutics are set to redefine the delivery of hypnotherapy. With the digital revolution sweeping across all sectors, including healthcare, the integration of technology in hypnotherapy presents an exciting frontier. Virtual Reality (VR) and Augmented Reality (AR) offer immersive experiences that could enhance the depth of hypnosis and its effectiveness. Dr David's interest in leveraging technology could see the development of VR-based hypnotherapy sessions, making the experience more vivid and impactful for clients across the globe.

Another significant area of development lies in Personalised Medicine and Genomics. As our understanding of the genetic basis of psychological conditions deepens, hypnotherapy could evolve to incorporate genetic insights, tailoring sessions more precisely to the individual's biological predispositions. This personalised approach would optimise therapeutic outcomes, resonating with Dr David's bespoke treatment plans, but with an added layer of genetic insight. Collaborative Care Models represent a holistic future direction, where hypnotherapy is integrated seamlessly with other forms of healthcare. Dr David's work in different cultural and clinical settings positions him uniquely to advocate for and develop integrative care models. These models could see hypnotherapy working hand in hand with traditional medical treatments, psychotherapy, and lifestyle interventions, offering a comprehensive approach to mental health and wellbeing.

Innovation in hypnotherapy, underpinned by rigorous research, is another area that promises to shape its future. Continuing to build an evidence base for the efficacy of hypnotherapy, particularly for conditions where traditional treatments have limited success, will be crucial. Dr David's commitment to evidence-based practice and continuous learning will undoubtedly contribute to this body of research, paving the way for hypnotherapy to gain broader acceptance and recognition in the medical community.

The future of hypnotherapy, with Dr David Postlethwaite steering its evolution, promises not only to uphold the profound legacy of this therapeutic modality but also to expand its boundaries, making it more effective, accessible, and integrated with the wider health care landscape.

How to Access Dr David's Hypnotherapy Sessions

Embarking on a journey of transformation with Dr David Postlethwaite is a straightforward process designed to accommodate individuals from various locations and walks of life. His reputation as a leading consultant hypnotherapist, coupled with a pioneering one-session model, has made his services highly sought after. To facilitate your initial step towards change, appointments can be conveniently scheduled through his official website. Here, you'll find detailed information on how to prepare for your session, alongside testimonials that attest to the efficacy of his unique approach.

For those preferring a more direct route, contacting his practice via telephone or email is an option. The responsive team is on hand to answer any queries you might have, from understanding the scope of issues Dr David can address to specifics about the session itself. They can also assist in arranging appointments that fit your schedule, ensuring a seamless and stress-free process.

Given the global reach of his expertise, Dr David also offers virtual sessions, breaking down geographical barriers and making his transformative hypnotherapy accessible to clients worldwide. This flexibility means that regardless of your location, Dr David's assistance is just a few clicks away.

Prior to your session, you will be guided through a preparatory phase to maximise the impact of your encounter with Dr David. This preparation is pivotal in tailoring the session to your specific needs, aligning with his philosophy of personalised care. Engaging with Dr David Postlethwaite's hypnotherapy sessions is an investment in your well-being, promising a personalised, empowering, and potentially life-altering experience.

Chapter 2

Hypnotherapy: Tracing its Origins from Ancient Greece to Today

Hypnotherapy is a practice that has been used for centuries to help individuals overcome various issues and improve their mental well-being. From its ancient roots in Greece to the pioneering work of modern practitioners like Dr. David Postlethwaite, hypnotherapy has a rich history that continues to evolve and grow. In this chapter, we will trace the origins of hypnotherapy from ancient Greece to the present day, exploring the key figures and developments that have shaped this fascinating field.

The Ancient Beginnings in Greece

Hypnotic practices have roots that reach deep into the annals of history, with the earliest recorded instances emanating from the ancient civilisation of Greece. It was here, amid the cradle of Western culture and philosophy, that the rudimentary forms of hypnotherapy were employed within the hallowed precincts of the Asclepieia. These sanctuaries, dedicated to Asclepius, the deity of medicine and healing, served as the nexus for therapeutic endeavours where sleep or trance-like states were induced as a part of the healing rituals.

Patients journeying to these temples in search of relief were led through a series of preparatory rituals, including purifications and the offering of sacrifices, before being guided into the abaton. This sacred space, often nestled within a darkened chamber, was where the incubation or temple sleep took place. It was believed that in these trance states, individuals could receive divine visions or messages, which the priests would later interpret to prescribe treatments, thus intertwining spiritual practice with therapeutic intervention.

The methodology employed in these ancient healing rites bears striking resemblance to modern hypnotherapy techniques. The focus on inducing a trance state to facilitate healing parallels contemporary hypnotherapy's use of hypnosis to access the subconscious mind, allowing for the treatment of both psychological and physical conditions. Additionally, the ancient Greeks' understanding of the interplay between the mind and body in these therapeutic contexts presaged the holistic approaches seen in today's hypnotherapy practices.

Moreover, the philosophical underpinnings of Greek society, with its emphasis on introspection and the exploration of the self, may have contributed to the development of these early hypnotic practices. Figures such as Pythagoras and Plato discussed concepts akin to the modern understanding of the unconscious mind, suggesting that these ideas were percolating through Greek thought long before they were formally recognised in the field of psychology.

These historical practices in Greece laid the foundational stones upon which the edifice of modern hypnotherapy was built. While the rituals and beliefs of ancient times have evolved, the essence of using altered states of consciousness to foster healing and well-being has remained a constant thread, weaving through the fabric of hypnotherapy's long and storied past.

The Influence of Franz Anton Mesmer

Franz Anton Mesmer, a figure of both intrigue and controversy in the 18th century, was pivotal in setting the stage for what would become hypnotherapy. Mesmer, originally from Germany, proposed the concept of "animal magnetism", a force he believed could heal the human body and was present in all living things. His methods, although unconventional, involved the use of magnets and his own hands to direct this supposed magnetic fluid in his patients' bodies, thereby inducing a trance-like state which he asserted could cure various ailments.

Mesmer's salons in Paris became the epicentres of his practice, where he would perform these treatments amidst an atmosphere charged with expectation and mystique. The theatricality of his methods, combined with the tangible effects observed in some of his patients, captured the public's imagination. However, it wasn't long before Mesmer's theories were scrutinised and criticised by the scientific community of the time. Despite this, the phenomenon he introduced—later termed "Mesmerism"—sowed the seeds for the future exploration of the mind's healing capabilities.

It's important to note that Mesmer's legacy is a complex one. His assertion that a natural energetic transference occurred between all objects in nature was met with scepticism, and his practices were largely discredited during his lifetime. Yet, the trance states he induced closely mimic what is recognised today as a hypnotic state. Mesmer's work indirectly challenged the medical and scientific communities to investigate the processes and potential of the mind more thoroughly, leading to a deeper understanding of psychological states and their impact on physical health.

Mesmer's contribution to the field of hypnotherapy, though initially mired in controversy, cannot be understated. His ability to induce altered states of consciousness in his patients opened the door to the therapeutic potential of trance states. The mesmerist movement he inspired persisted well into the 19th century, influencing practitioners across Europe and America, and setting the groundwork for the formal scientific investigation of hypnosis by figures such as James Braid.

In essence, Franz Anton Mesmer was a catalyst for change. His work compelled the medical world to explore the connection between the mind and body more closely, laying the foundational principles that would evolve into the practice of hypnotherapy as it is known today. Although the theory of animal magnetism has been relegated to the annals of pseudoscience, Mesmer's impact on the development of therapeutic hypnosis remains a testament to his influential, if controversial, legacy.

James Braid and the Birth of Hypnotherapy

The journey of hypnotherapy witnessed a significant turning point in the 19th century with the advent of James Braid, a Scottish surgeon whose curiosity and scientific approach to what was then known as 'mesmerism' led to a pivotal transformation in the understanding and application of hypnosis. Distancing himself from the mystical connotations associated with Franz Anton Mesmer's work, Braid sought to establish a more rational and empirical framework for the hypnotic process. His investigations marked the genesis of hypnotherapy as a scientifically grounded practice.

Braid's initial encounter with the phenomenon of mesmerism was one of scepticism. However, upon witnessing firsthand the effects of what he would later term 'hypnosis', he became convinced of its potential therapeutic benefits. Unlike Mesmer, who attributed the effects of his treatments to a quasi-mystical fluid, Braid proposed that the hypnotic state was induced through focused attention and was a result of psychological and physiological processes.

In 1843, Braid introduced the term 'neuro-hypnotism' (nervous sleep) to describe this state, later shortening it to 'hypnosis', after Hypnos, the Greek god of sleep. Although his terminology suggested a sleep-like condition, Braid believed hypnosis to be a form of heightened concentration that enabled direct communication with the subconscious mind. This concept laid the foundation for hypnotherapy, distinguishing it from the mesmerist practices of the past.

Braid's contributions extended beyond mere nomenclature. He meticulously documented his observations and developed techniques for inducing hypnosis, demonstrating its application in pain management, especially in dentistry and minor surgeries at a time when anaesthetics were not yet widely available. His work presented hypnosis as a viable and beneficial tool in therapeutic settings, paving the way for its acceptance in medical and psychological communities.

Through public lectures and writings, such as his seminal work, 'Neurypnology or the Rationale of Nervous Sleep', Braid worked tirelessly to demystify hypnosis and advocate for its scientific investigation. His efforts to reframe hypnosis in the context of medical science were instrumental in changing perceptions of the practice, enabling its evolution into the hypnotherapy used in contemporary therapeutic settings.

Braid's legacy in the realm of hypnotherapy is profound. By grounding hypnosis in the science of the mind and body, he not only revolutionised how it was perceived but also expanded its potential as a tool for healing, laying the groundwork for the development of modern hypnotherapy.

Sigmund Freud's Exploration of the Unconscious
Sigmund Freud, the father of psychoanalysis, ventured into the depths of the human psyche, unravelling the complexities of the unconscious mind. His foray into hypnotherapy, albeit brief, was a period marked by insightful exploration into the therapeutic potentials of accessing the unconscious. Freud's engagement with hypnosis began in the late 19th century, influenced by his interactions with renowned figures in the field, such as Jean-Martin Charcot and Josef Breuer. These experiences laid the groundwork for his subsequent theoretical developments.

Freud initially utilised hypnosis as a means to explore the unconscious thoughts and feelings of his patients, believing that the hypnotic state provided a gateway to the deeper recesses of the mind that were otherwise inaccessible. Through these hypnotic sessions, he observed the emergence of repressed memories and unresolved conflicts, reinforcing his theory that the unconscious mind plays a significant role in shaping human behaviour and psychological disorders.

However, Freud's relationship with hypnosis was complex and evolving. He encountered limitations with the technique, particularly its variability in effectiveness among patients. Some were highly susceptible to hypnotic induction, whilst others remained impervious. This inconsistency, coupled with his growing interest in the power of free association and dream analysis, led Freud to gradually shift away from hypnotherapy. He developed the talking cure, or psychoanalysis, as an alternative approach to accessing the unconscious mind, without the need for hypnotic trance.

Despite distancing himself from hypnotherapy, Freud's early work contributed significantly to the field. His emphasis on the unconscious as a source of psychological distress and his exploratory techniques informed later developments in hypnotherapy. Freud's legacy in hypnotherapy is embodied in the principle that unlocking the unconscious can provide profound insights and pathways to healing. His pioneering efforts underscored the importance of the unconscious in therapeutic practice, a concept that remains integral to various forms of hypnotherapy and psychotherapeutic techniques today.

Freud's explorations into the unconscious through hypnosis, although a chapter in his broader journey towards psychoanalysis, highlighted the therapeutic value of engaging with the hidden aspects of the psyche. This acknowledgement of the unconscious as a terrain ripe for therapeutic intervention paved the way for more nuanced and sophisticated approaches to mental health treatment, influencing generations of practitioners and shaping the trajectory of hypnotherapy and psychotherapy alike.

The 20th Century and Hypnotherapy's Growing Acceptance
The evolution of hypnotherapy throughout the 20th century marks a period of significant progress and wider recognition within the medical and psychological fields. This era witnessed the transformation of hypnotherapy from a fringe element, often associated with mysticism and scepticism, into a respected therapeutic practice. The growing body of empirical research, along with a better understanding of the psychological underpinnings of the mind and behaviour, played a crucial role in this transition.
As the century progressed, notable figures emerged who contributed to the scientific exploration and application of hypnotherapy. These practitioners and researchers worked diligently to establish a more robust theoretical framework for hypnosis, moving away from the mystical explanations of the past and grounding their findings in observable and measurable outcomes. The publication of scholarly articles and clinical studies provided evidence of the efficacy of hypnotherapy in treating a myriad of conditions, from anxiety and depression to pain management and behavioural change, further solidifying its legitimacy.

Moreover, the integration of hypnotherapy into broader therapeutic modalities highlighted its versatility and effectiveness as a complementary treatment. Psychotherapists began to incorporate hypnotic techniques into their sessions, utilising the heightened state of suggestibility to facilitate deeper introspection and change. This period also saw the establishment of professional bodies and societies dedicated to the study and practice of hypnotherapy, setting standards for training and ethical practice, which were instrumental in its professionalisation.

The increasing acceptance of hypnotherapy was further evidenced by its use in medical settings, particularly in anaesthesiology, where it served as an adjunct to conventional anaesthetic techniques or as a standalone method in cases of allergy to anaesthetic drugs. Its application in easing the psychological and physical discomfort of childbirth and dental procedures demonstrated hypnotherapy's broad applicability and acceptance.

The latter part of the 20th century also witnessed the advent of more nuanced approaches, such as cognitive-behavioural hypnotherapy, which combines cognitive-behavioural therapy with hypnotherapeutic methods to achieve more effective outcomes. This blending of approaches underscored the adaptive nature of hypnotherapy and its capacity to evolve in line with advancements in psychological sciences.

In sum, the 20th century heralded a new era for hypnotherapy, characterised by scientific inquiry, professionalisation, and a growing recognition of its value as a therapeutic tool. This period laid the groundwork for the contemporary practice of hypnotherapy, paving the way for innovative developments and the expansion of its applications in health and well-being.

Dr. David Postlethwaite's Modern Contributions

In the ever-evolving landscape of hypnotherapy, Dr. David Postlethwaite emerges as a contemporary figure whose work has significantly impacted the discipline. Building upon the rich tapestry of hypnotherapy's history, Dr. Postlethwaite has propelled the practice into the modern era with innovative approaches and a deep understanding of its therapeutic potential. His contributions, particularly through groundbreaking books and the development of downloadable hypnotherapy sessions, have revolutionised the way individuals engage with and benefit from hypnotherapy.

Dr. Postlethwaite's expertise and dedication to the field have led to the creation of a suite of resources that cater to a diverse range of issues, from anxiety and stress to smoking cessation and weight loss. These resources, characterised by their accessibility and efficacy, reflect his commitment to making hypnotherapy a readily available tool for personal development and healing. His approach combines traditional hypnotherapeutic techniques with the insights of modern psychology, offering a comprehensive and holistic method to address the complexities of the human psyche.

The downloadable sessions, a hallmark of Dr. Postlethwaite's work, represent a significant advancement in the practice of hypnotherapy. By harnessing the power of digital technology, these sessions provide a flexible and user-friendly option for individuals seeking to explore the benefits of hypnotherapy from the comfort of their own homes. This innovation not only democratises access to hypnotherapy but also aligns with contemporary lifestyles, where digital solutions are increasingly favoured for health and well-being interventions.

Beyond the practical applications of his work, Dr. Postlethwaite's contributions to the theoretical underpinnings of hypnotherapy have also been noteworthy. His publications delve into the scientific principles behind hypnosis, offering readers a grounded understanding of its mechanisms and potential. Through his writings, he advocates for a nuanced appreciation of hypnotherapy, encouraging both practitioners and clients to recognise its value as a legitimate and effective therapeutic modality.

As hypnotherapy continues to gain prominence in the fields of psychology and healthcare, the work of Dr. David Postlethwaite stands as a testament to the potential for innovation within traditional therapeutic frameworks. His modern contributions not only enrich the practice of hypnotherapy but also ensure its relevance and accessibility for future generations.

The Science Behind Hypnotherapy Today

Contemporary research into hypnotherapy has illuminated its capacity to influence both the mind and body, uncovering the intricate science that underpins its efficacy. With advancements in neuroscience, we now have greater insight into how hypnosis affects neural activity, allowing us to better understand the physiological and psychological shifts that occur during a hypnotic trance. Studies employing functional magnetic resonance imaging (fMRI) and electroencephalogram (EEG) technologies have revealed distinct changes in brain wave patterns, demonstrating a heightened state of concentration and suggestibility that defines the hypnotic state.

This scientific exploration has also extended to the realm of psychoneuroimmunology, where research suggests that hypnotherapy can modulate immune function and stress responses, offering potential pathways for treating autoimmune disorders and chronic stress-related conditions. The application of hypnotherapy has been shown to lead to measurable changes in the body, such as reduced pain perception, lowered blood pressure, and improved gastrointestinal function, indicating its utility as a non-pharmacological intervention in healthcare.

Moreover, the cognitive-behavioural framework has been enriched by integrating hypnotherapeutic techniques, facilitating deeper insights into how thoughts and beliefs can influence emotional and physical health. This approach has led to the development of targeted interventions for a variety of conditions, from phobias and anxiety disorders to sleep disturbances and addiction, showcasing the versatility and depth of hypnotherapy as a therapeutic modality.

The ongoing investigation into the mechanisms of action behind hypnotherapy not only reinforces its legitimacy as a scientific practice but also enhances its effectiveness as a treatment option. As research continues to unfold, it is anticipated that our comprehension of hypnosis will deepen, leading to more refined and potent therapeutic techniques that capitalise on the complex interplay between the mind, brain, and body. The current trajectory of hypnotherapy research promises to expand its applications and improve its integration into mainstream healthcare, ensuring that it remains a vital component of psychological and medical interventions.

Hypnotherapy in the Digital Age
The digital revolution has significantly transformed the landscape of hypnotherapy, ushering in a new era of accessibility and convenience for individuals worldwide. In today's interconnected world, the power of hypnotherapy can be tapped into from the comfort of one's own home, thanks to the proliferation of online resources and mobile applications. This digital evolution has not only democratised access to hypnotherapy but also tailored it to fit the fast-paced and varied lifestyles of the modern populace.

Online platforms and bespoke apps now offer an extensive array of hypnotherapy sessions, covering a broad spectrum of needs - from stress relief and anxiety management to smoking cessation and weight control. These digital offerings are designed to provide users with the flexibility to engage in therapeutic sessions at times and places that suit them best, breaking down the barriers of time and geography that previously limited access to traditional face-to-face therapy.

Moreover, the quality and effectiveness of these digital hypnotherapy solutions have been bolstered by advancements in audio and visual technologies. High-quality, immersive audio recordings guide individuals into deep states of relaxation and suggestibility, mirroring the experience of in-person sessions. Additionally, interactive features and personalised session pathways offer a customised therapeutic experience, catering to the unique needs and preferences of each user.

The shift towards digital hypnotherapy has also facilitated a greater level of privacy and anonymity, which can be particularly appealing for those who may feel apprehensive about seeking help. The ability to explore and utilise hypnotherapy discreetly encourages more individuals to take the first step towards mental well-being.

Importantly, the rise of digital hypnotherapy has prompted a surge in the availability of evidence-based and professionally produced content. Renowned practitioners, such as Dr. David Postlethwaite, have extended their reach through downloadable sessions and online materials, ensuring that users have access to reputable and effective therapeutic tools. This blending of professional expertise with digital convenience represents a significant milestone in the field of hypnotherapy, promising to further its impact and efficacy.

As we move forward, the digitalisation of hypnotherapy stands as a beacon of innovation and progress, making profound healing and self-improvement more attainable than ever before. The marriage of technology and traditional therapeutic techniques marks a pivotal chapter in the ongoing story of hypnotherapy, highlighting its adaptability and enduring relevance in the digital age.

Chapter 3

Using Hypnotherapy to Solve Life's Challenges: A Comprehensive Guide

Hypnotherapy has been gaining popularity as a powerful tool to help individuals overcome a variety of challenges in their lives. Whether it's dealing with anxiety, breaking bad habits, or even addressing phobias, hypnotherapy has shown to be effective in helping people make positive changes. In this comprehensive guide, we will explore the various ways in which a competent degree qualified hypnotherapist can assist individuals in overcoming life's obstacles.

Overcoming Anxiety and Stress with Hypnotherapy

In today's fast-paced world, the prevalence of anxiety and stress is higher than ever, affecting a significant proportion of the population. Hypnotherapy presents a promising avenue for those seeking relief from these pervasive issues. By engaging the mind in a state of heightened awareness and focus, a degree-qualified hypnotherapist can facilitate profound and lasting changes in the way individuals respond to anxiety-inducing situations.

The process begins with the hypnotherapist guiding the client into a deeply relaxed state, where the conscious mind takes a step back, allowing direct communication with the subconscious. It is within this state that the hypnotherapist can uncover the underlying causes of the client's anxiety and stress. Often, these emotions stem from past experiences or ingrained beliefs that the individual may not even be consciously aware of. Through careful exploration and gentle guidance, these root causes can be identified and addressed.

A key technique used in hypnotherapy for managing anxiety and stress is the use of positive suggestions. These suggestions are crafted to counteract negative thought patterns and beliefs that contribute to the client's distress. By embedding these positive affirmations into the subconscious, the individual can start to experience shifts in their perception, leading to a reduction in anxiety levels and an improved ability to handle stress.

Visualisation is another powerful tool employed by hypnotherapists. Clients are encouraged to envisage themselves successfully navigating situations that would typically trigger anxiety or stress. This mental rehearsal helps to build confidence and resilience, equipping individuals with the skills to face challenges with a sense of calm and control.
Moreover, hypnotherapy empowers clients to develop new coping mechanisms. Techniques such as deep breathing, mindfulness, and self-hypnosis are often taught, providing individuals with practical strategies to manage stress and anxiety in their day-to-day lives. By learning to access their inner resources, clients can cultivate a more peaceful and balanced state of mind.

In essence, hypnotherapy offers a pathway to transforming the way individuals experience and respond to anxiety and stress. Through the therapeutic partnership with a skilled hypnotherapist, clients can achieve significant improvements in their mental well-being, leading to a more fulfilling and stress-free life.

Hypnotherapy's Role in Treating Depression
Depression is a complex condition that extends its reach deeply into an individual's life, manifesting through a myriad of symptoms including persistent sadness, lack of interest in previously enjoyable activities, and an overwhelming sense of hopelessness. Where traditional treatments may not suffice alone, hypnotherapy emerges as a complementary approach, offering a beacon of hope for those grappling with this debilitating condition.

A degree-qualified hypnotherapist can delve into the subconscious mind, the arena where negative thought cycles and patterns reside and exert their influence. By establishing a connection with this part of the mind, the therapist can introduce new, positive constructs that challenge and alter the negative beliefs underpinning depression. This process is akin to planting seeds of optimism in fertile ground, where they can grow and flourish, gradually reshaping the individual's mental landscape towards a more positive and hopeful outlook.

In sessions tailored to addressing depression, the hypnotherapist utilises a blend of techniques designed to foster a change in the emotional and cognitive processes of the client. One such method is the use of metaphor and storytelling, which can facilitate a deeper understanding and internalisation of positive concepts and attitudes. These narratives speak directly to the subconscious, bypassing the critical conscious mind, to instigate meaningful and lasting change.

Guided imagery is another cornerstone of hypnotherapy for depression. Clients are led through vivid, positive experiences in their mind's eye, which can help to lighten the pervasive darkness of depression. These guided visualisations are not merely escapist fantasies but serve as rehearsals for real-life experiences of joy, accomplishment, and contentment, gradually diminishing the hold of depressive symptoms.

Furthermore, the therapeutic journey through hypnotherapy often uncovers and addresses the root causes of depression, whether they are past traumas, unresolved conflicts, or ingrained beliefs about self-worth. By bringing these to light and reprocessing them in a supportive and healing environment, individuals can make peace with their past and forge a path towards recovery.

Hypnotherapy, in its essence, offers more than just a coping mechanism for depression; it provides a transformative experience that can rekindle hope, renew interest in life, and restore the joy of living. Through the dedicated guidance of a degree-qualified hypnotherapist, individuals find not only relief from the symptoms of depression but also embark on a profound journey towards healing and self-rediscovery.

Breaking Bad Habits Through Hypnotherapy

Habits, whether smoking, habitual overeating, or incessant nail-biting, often serve as coping mechanisms for underlying stress or emotional discomfort. Breaking free from these ingrained patterns requires more than just willpower; it necessitates a profound transformation in the subconscious drivers of behaviour. This is where hypnotherapy, guided by a degree-qualified practitioner, comes into play, offering a tailored approach to habit cessation.

A key aspect of hypnotherapy in habit breaking is its ability to pinpoint and address the root causes of unwanted behaviour. For many, these habits have become deeply embedded responses to certain triggers, whether emotional, situational, or environmental. Through hypnotherapy, individuals can uncover these triggers, understand their origins, and develop new, healthier coping strategies. The hypnotherapist facilitates this process by guiding the individual into a state of deep relaxation, wherein the subconscious mind becomes more accessible and receptive to positive change.

The power of suggestion plays a pivotal role in this therapeutic journey. During sessions, the hypnotherapist introduces carefully crafted suggestions that resonate with the individual's desire to break the habit. These suggestions are designed to recalibrate subconscious thought patterns, diminishing the habit's hold and reinforcing the individual's commitment to change. By replacing negative behaviours with positive affirmations, the individual begins to forge a new self-image, one that is free from the constraints of past habits.

Visualisation techniques further enhance the effectiveness of hypnotherapy in breaking bad habits. Clients are encouraged to visualise themselves successfully overcoming temptations and living a life unburdened by their previous compulsions. These visualisations not only instil a sense of achievement but also prepare the mind for real-world success, reinforcing the belief that change is not only possible but imminent.

In essence, hypnotherapy offers a holistic and personalised path to habit change, engaging both the mind and emotions in the pursuit of well-being. By addressing the psychological underpinnings of bad habits and fostering a positive mindset, a degree-qualified hypnotherapist can empower individuals to transcend their limitations and embrace a healthier, more fulfilling lifestyle.

Addressing Phobias and Fears with Hypnotherapy

Phobias and fears, whether of heights, flying, or spiders, can deeply limit a person's ability to live their life fully. These intense fears often stem from past experiences or learned behaviours and can seem insurmountable to those who suffer from them. However, through the intervention of a degree-qualified hypnotherapist, individuals can find a way to navigate through these fears and reclaim their freedom.

The process begins with the hypnotherapist establishing a safe and supportive environment where the client can explore the origins of their fear. This understanding is crucial, as it allows the therapy to be tailored specifically to the individual's needs. Through guided relaxation, the client is brought into a state of heightened suggestibility, where they are more open to positive influences and changes in perception.

One of the most effective techniques used in hypnotherapy for phobias is systematic desensitisation. This involves the gradual and controlled exposure to the object or situation that causes fear, all within the safety of the hypnotic state. By confronting their fear in a controlled manner, the client can begin to dissociate the object of their phobia from the automatic fear response it triggers.

Visualisation techniques also play a pivotal role. Clients are guided to visualise themselves handling situations involving their phobia with calmness and confidence. These positive visualisations help to build a new framework within the subconscious, one where the fear is no longer in control. Instead, the client is able to see themselves as capable and in charge, significantly reducing the power the phobia has over them.

Additionally, hypnotherapy can instil new coping strategies, equipping individuals with the tools to manage their response when faced with situations that previously would have triggered fear. This empowerment is a key aspect of the therapeutic process, enabling clients to approach previously feared situations with a new sense of confidence and control.

Through these methods, hypnotherapy offers a pathway to overcoming phobias and fears, allowing individuals to lead richer, more fulfilling lives without the constraints imposed by irrational fears.

Hypnotherapy in Pain Management

Chronic pain, a widespread affliction affecting countless individuals worldwide, presents a significant barrier to the enjoyment of everyday activities and overall life satisfaction. In the quest for relief, many are turning to hypnotherapy, a method that stands out for its gentle, non-pharmacological approach. This form of therapy, guided by a degree-qualified hypnotherapist, taps into the profound connection between the mind and the body, offering a pathway to pain reduction that is rooted in the power of the subconscious.

The journey towards managing pain with hypnotherapy begins with the therapist helping the client to achieve a state of deep relaxation. Within this state, individuals become more receptive to positive suggestions and healing imagery, which are pivotal in altering the perception of pain. The subconscious mind, now accessible and open, can be encouraged to perceive pain differently, potentially reducing its intensity and the emotional distress associated with it.

One of the core techniques utilised in this form of therapy is visualisation. Clients are guided to imagine themselves in scenarios where they are free from pain, or where the pain is manageable and does not interfere with their quality of life. This mental imagery not only distracts from the immediate sensation of pain but also reprograms the mind to deal with discomfort in a more constructive manner.

Moreover, hypnotherapy aids in identifying and addressing any psychological factors that may be exacerbating the pain. Stress, anxiety, and depression are known to intensify pain perception; hence, by tackling these issues, a hypnotherapist can indirectly contribute to pain relief. Additionally, clients are often equipped with self-hypnosis techniques, enabling them to tap into their newly learned coping strategies whenever needed, thus fostering a sense of control and autonomy over their condition.

In essence, hypnotherapy for pain management is a testament to the therapeutic potential of accessing and influencing the subconscious mind. It offers individuals a means to not only alleviate physical discomfort but also to empower them with the tools to enhance their mental and emotional resilience in the face of chronic pain.

Enhancing Performance Through Hypnotherapy

Performance anxiety and related issues can significantly obstruct one's potential in various domains such as sport, academia, and the professional environment. Hypnotherapy emerges as an effective solution to navigate through these impediments, unlocking the individual's innate capacity for excellence. With the guidance of a degree-qualified hypnotherapist, individuals can embark on a transformative journey, redefining their approach towards performance-related challenges.

The process utilises the therapeutic power of the subconscious mind to reshape one's self-perception and eliminate the mental barriers to success. A common method employed in these sessions involves the strategic use of positive affirmations and suggestions tailored to bolster confidence and self-belief. By embedding these constructive messages into the subconscious, clients gradually adopt a more assured and optimistic outlook towards their abilities.

Visualisation plays a crucial role in enhancing performance through hypnotherapy. Clients are guided to vividly imagine achieving their goals, be it delivering a flawless presentation, excelling in a sporting event, or surpassing academic expectations. These mental rehearsals not only prepare the individual for the task at hand but also instil a sense of preparedness and calm, essential components for peak performance.

Another facet of this approach is addressing the root causes of performance anxiety. Through hypnotherapy, individuals can explore and understand the underlying factors contributing to their fears and apprehensions. This deep level of insight allows for a more nuanced intervention, where specific anxieties can be targeted and alleviated, clearing the path for enhanced focus and concentration.

By fostering a mindset geared towards success, hypnotherapy equips individuals with the mental tools necessary to overcome the psychological hurdles that hinder performance. The result is an empowered individual, capable of tapping into their full potential and excelling in their chosen field. Through the expert support of a hypnotherapist, clients learn to harness the power of their subconscious, transforming performance anxiety into an opportunity for growth and achievement.

Hypnotherapy for Sleep Disorders
In the realm of sleep disorders, where individuals often find themselves trapped in a cycle of restless nights and weary days, hypnotherapy emerges as a beacon of hope. Facilitated by a degree-qualified hypnotherapist, this therapeutic approach delves deep into the subconscious mind to unlock patterns and behaviours that inhibit healthy sleep.

The journey towards improved sleep through hypnotherapy begins with identifying and addressing the root causes that disrupt sleep, such as anxiety, stress, or deep-seated fears. Unlike conventional treatments that might only skim the surface, hypnotherapy seeks to resolve these underlying issues, paving the way for a lasting solution to sleep disturbances.

A pivotal technique within this process is the cultivation of a deeply relaxed state. Here, the individual is guided away from the tumult of conscious worries and into a serene mental space. This shift is critical, as it allows the mind to embrace positive suggestions tailored to foster good sleep hygiene. These suggestions are carefully designed to recalibrate the subconscious's perception of bedtime routines, transforming them from sources of stress into triggers for relaxation and sleep.

Visualisation exercises are another cornerstone of this approach. Clients are encouraged to envision themselves drifting effortlessly into a deep, restorative sleep, night after night. This practice not only prepares the mind for the act of sleeping but also reinforces the belief in the individual's ability to achieve uninterrupted rest.

Additionally, hypnotherapy empowers clients with techniques for self-guided relaxation, enabling them to independently manage and mitigate instances of insomnia. Through repeated sessions, individuals learn to harness these strategies, gradually diminishing their reliance on external aids for sleep.

The integration of hypnotherapy into the management of sleep disorders offers more than just a temporary reprieve; it equips individuals with the tools and insights necessary for long-term improvement. By aligning the subconscious with positive sleep patterns, hypnotherapy holds the potential to significantly enhance the quality of life, allowing the nights to be a time of peaceful restoration once more.

The Role of Hypnotherapy in Weight Management
Navigating the journey of weight management often requires more than just adjustments to diet and exercise; it demands a deep dive into the psychological underpinnings that fuel our eating habits and lifestyle choices. This is where the expertise of a degree-qualified hypnotherapist can be transformative, offering a nuanced approach to achieving and maintaining a healthy weight.

At the heart of hypnotherapy's role in weight management is its capacity to uncover and address the subconscious drivers behind unhealthy eating patterns. These may include emotional eating, where food serves as a source of comfort during stress or sadness, or ingrained beliefs about food stemming from childhood. By bringing these hidden motivators into the light, hypnotherapy enables individuals to understand and overcome the barriers to their weight loss success.

The therapeutic process typically involves guiding the client into a relaxed state, where the subconscious mind becomes more open to suggestion. Within this receptive state, the hypnotherapist introduces positive affirmations designed to shift attitudes towards food and self-image. These affirmations encourage a move away from harmful patterns towards behaviours that support well-being and weight management goals.

Another key aspect is the development of a healthier relationship with food. Through hypnotherapy, individuals learn to listen to their body's cues for hunger and fullness, breaking free from the cycle of overeating and guilt. The focus shifts from short-term dieting to long-term lifestyle changes, fostering a sense of control and empowerment.

Moreover, hypnotherapy can enhance motivation for physical activity, embedding the desire for movement into one's daily routine. By visualising the outcomes they wish to achieve, clients can cultivate a positive mindset that underpins their efforts towards weight management.

In essence, hypnotherapy offers a comprehensive approach to weight management, addressing the psychological, emotional, and behavioural aspects. It equips individuals with the tools to rewrite their narrative around food and exercise, paving the way for lasting change and a healthier, more balanced life.

Hypnotherapy and the Journey to Self-Discovery
The profound journey towards self-discovery is uniquely facilitated by the practices of hypnotherapy, offering a window into the deepest layers of one's psyche. Through the skilled guidance of a degree-qualified hypnotherapist, individuals embark on an explorative quest that illuminates the intricacies of their inner world, revealing insights that were previously obscured or unacknowledged. This

exploration fosters an enriched understanding of personal values, beliefs, and the underlying motives driving behaviour, thereby paving the way for significant personal growth and development.

In the therapeutic setting, the individual is gently led into a state of deep relaxation, a process which lowers the barriers to the subconscious mind, making it receptive to introspection and self-reflection. Within this tranquil mental space, the individual can confront and reconcile with aspects of their self-identity that may be contributing to internal conflicts or emotional turmoil. Hypnotherapy assists in unearthing these hidden elements, facilitating a process of healing and integration.

The application of tailored suggestions and visualisation techniques further enhances this journey, enabling individuals to envisage their ideal self and the manifestation of their core values in their daily lives. Such practices not only affirm one's aspirations but also instil a profound sense of self-belief and empowerment, critical for personal transformation.

Ultimately, hypnotherapy stands as a beacon for those seeking to deepen their understanding of themselves, offering a compassionate and empowering route to self-discovery. It encourages an alignment with one's true self, leading to a life lived with greater authenticity, purpose, and fulfilment.

Chapter 4

Dr Postlethwaite's hypnotherapy downloads offer a convenient and scientifically backed approach to improving your well-being from the comfort of your own home.

Unveiling the Power of Hypnotherapy

Hypnotherapy, often shrouded in mystery and misconceptions, is in fact a clinically validated practice that has garnered scientific support for its efficacy in treating a broad spectrum of conditions. At its core, hypnotherapy is a therapeutic technique that utilises hypnosis to induce a state of focused attention and heightened suggestibility. Within this trance-like state, individuals are more open to suggestions and interventions that can catalyse profound changes in behaviour, emotions, and the physical state.

The mechanism behind hypnotherapy is rooted in its ability to access the subconscious mind. This part of our brain operates below the level of conscious awareness, influencing a wide array of behaviours and responses. Traditional therapeutic approaches primarily engage the conscious mind and are sometimes unable to bypass the deeply ingrained patterns residing within the subconscious. Hypnotherapy, however, directly engages with this inner realm, facilitating more effective and lasting transformations.

Critically, the scientific community has begun to unravel the workings of hypnotherapy through rigorous research. Neuroimaging studies have illustrated how hypnotherapy can alter brain activity in ways that correlate with reduced pain perception, anxiety, and stress levels, among other benefits. These findings lend credence to the practice and explain why hypnotherapy has become a sought-after treatment for managing conditions such as chronic pain, sleep disorders, and various forms of addiction.

This therapeutic power also lies in its versatility. By tailoring suggestions and therapeutic goals to the individual's specific needs, hypnotherapy can be adapted to support a wide array of personal objectives. Whether it's bolstering self-esteem, overcoming behavioural challenges, or mitigating the impacts of trauma, hypnotherapy holds the potential to unlock personal growth and healing.

In the hands of a skilled practitioner like Dr David Postlethwaite, hypnotherapy transcends its misconceptions to reveal a scientifically backed pathway to wellness. With a deep understanding of the subconscious mind and a nuanced approach to individual care, Dr Postlethwaite harnesses the full spectrum of hypnotherapy's potential. His extensive experience not only ensures a safe and supportive environment for transformation but also amplifies the effectiveness of each session, paving the way for meaningful, long-term change.

Thus, unveiling the power of hypnotherapy reveals it as not just an alternative therapy but as a scientifically endorsed avenue for personal evolution, offering hope and healing to those who may feel they have exhausted other options.
Dr Postlethwaite's Expertise and Approach

Navigating the realms of mental and emotional wellness, Dr David Postlethwaite stands as a beacon of expertise and insight in the field of hypnotherapy. With an impressive tenure exceeding three decades as a consultant hypnotherapist, Dr Postlethwaite's approach is steeped in both science and the nuanced understanding of individual experiences. His practice is not just about the application of hypnotherapy techniques; it is an embodiment of compassion, dedication, and an unwavering commitment to personalised care.

Dr Postlethwaite's methodology is distinct in its foundation on empirical evidence and its alignment with the latest advancements in psychological research. This evidence-based approach ensures that every hypnotherapy session is more than a mere exercise in relaxation—it's a scientifically grounded endeavour aimed at effecting tangible change. By meticulously integrating the science of the subconscious with the art of therapeutic suggestion, he crafts interventions that resonate deeply with the core of individual issues.

A cornerstone of Dr Postlethwaite's practice is the establishment of a safe and supportive therapeutic environment. The journey into the subconscious can be intimate and, for some, daunting. Dr Postlethwaite is acutely aware of these dynamics and prioritises creating a space where clients feel entirely at ease to explore their inner worlds. This sense of security and trust is crucial, as it fosters an openness to the therapeutic process and enhances receptivity to transformative suggestions.

The holistic approach championed by Dr Postlethwaite extends beyond addressing specific issues; it is aimed at nurturing overall wellbeing and empowering individuals towards sustained self-improvement. His expertise and approach are not just about facilitating temporary relief but about igniting a journey of self-discovery, healing, and profound personal growth.

In an era where the quest for mental health solutions is ever-pressing, Dr David Postlethwaite's hypnotherapy practice offers a beacon of hope and transformation.

The Science Behind the Sessions

The underlying science of Dr Postlethwaite's hypnotherapy sessions draws upon a fascinating interplay between the conscious and subconscious minds. Hypnotherapy's efficacy is increasingly supported by a growing body of neuroscientific research, revealing its potential to enact profound and lasting changes in mental and physical health. Neuroimaging studies, for instance, have provided compelling evidence of the ways hypnotherapy can modify brain activity, shedding light on its ability to alleviate pain, reduce symptoms of anxiety, and diminish stress.

The process hinges on the principle of neuroplasticity, the profound personal evolution. Individuals embarking on the journey with Dr Postlethwaite's hypnotherapy downloads have discovered avenues of change that once seemed unreachable. Through the nuanced application of hypnotherapeutic techniques, barriers that have long impeded personal growth and wellbeing are dismantled, allowing for an emergence of new, empowering narratives.
The stories of transformation are as diverse as the individuals themselves. For some, the relief from the grip of chronic pain marks the beginning of a newfound freedom, enabling engagement with life's pleasures that were previously marred by discomfort. Others find solace in the quieting of anxiety's persistent whisper, a change that opens doors to confidence and the embrace of opportunities once avoided. The recalibration of sleep patterns stands out for many as a turning point, where the restoration of restful nights lays the foundation for more vibrant, energetic days.

But the impact of hypnotherapy, particularly under the guidance of Dr Postlethwaite, is not confined to these tangible benefits. The shifts experienced resonate on a deeper level, influencing one's self-perception and interaction with the world. The journey towards smoking cessation or the moderation of eating behaviours, for example, often unveils underlying layers of self-esteem and control, illuminating paths towards broader personal empowerment. The success stories extend into the realm of emotional resilience, where individuals learn to navigate the turbulence of life's challenges with grace and fortitude, transforming their responses to stress and adversity.

Moreover, the process itself embodies an act of self-care and commitment to one's mental health, reinforcing the understanding that personal wellbeing is both a right and a responsibility. This realisation is, in itself, life-changing, fostering a mindset oriented towards continuous self-improvement and wellbeing.

As individuals traverse these paths of change, the common thread that binds their experiences is the discovery of their own capacity for self-directed change. The realisation that the power to transform lies within, unlocked by the guiding hand of hypnotherapy, is perhaps the most profound impact of all. In this light, Dr Postlethwaite's hypnotherapy downloads do not just offer a solution to immediate concerns; they unlock the door to a lifetime of potential and personal mastery.

The Convenience of At-Home Hypnotherapy Downloads

In today's fast-paced world, finding time for self-care and mental health can be a challenge. The beauty of Dr Postlethwaite's hypnotherapy downloads lies in their seamless integration into your daily routine, allowing for therapeutic intervention without the need for disruptive scheduling or travel to a clinic. This convenience ensures that individuals can engage with hypnotherapy sessions at a time and place that suits them best, be it during a quiet morning, a lunch break, or in the tranquil moments before sleep.

The digital format of these downloads demystifies the process of hypnotherapy, making it accessible and manageable. There's an innate flexibility that comes with having these therapeutic tools at your fingertips, ready to be used as often as needed. This adaptability not only caters to various lifestyles and commitments but also allows for repetition of sessions, reinforcing their benefits and enhancing their effectiveness over time.

Furthermore, the privacy afforded by at-home hypnotherapy downloads can be particularly appealing. For those who may feel apprehensive about undergoing hypnosis in a traditional face-to-face setting, the discretion provided by this modality can encourage a willingness to explore hypnotherapy without the perceived stigma or vulnerability. This aspect is crucial, as comfort and openness are key to maximising the therapeutic experience.

Dr Postlethwaite's expertly crafted sessions offer a bridge to wellness that respects the complexities of modern life. They encapsulate a sophisticated understanding of hypnotherapy's principles while delivering them in a format that resonates with the needs of today's individuals seeking mental health support. The ease with which these sessions can be incorporated into daily life enhances their appeal, breaking down barriers to mental health care and fostering a culture of wellness that is both inclusive and adaptable.

By eliminating the obstacles traditionally associated with seeking therapy, Dr Postlethwaite's hypnotherapy downloads represent a forward-thinking approach to mental health. They affirm the notion that access to transformative psychological support can and should be as uncomplicated and as unintrusive as possible, paving the way for a more balanced, healthier existence for those who choose to embark on this journey.

Tailoring the Experience to Your Needs
In the realm of personal growth and healing, the importance of a tailored approach cannot be overstated. Recognising that each individual's path is marked by distinct challenges and goals, Dr Postlethwaite's hypnotherapy downloads have been meticulously designed to cater to a wide spectrum of needs. This bespoke nature of the therapy sessions ensures that they resonate deeply with the person at their core, facilitating a more impactful and enduring transformation.

The spectrum of downloads available encompasses a range of objectives, from alleviating anxiety and stress to fostering better sleep patterns and boosting self-esteem. This variety ensures that whether you are seeking to overcome a specific hurdle or to enhance your overall well-being, there is a session calibrated to your precise requirements. The beauty of this customisation lies in its ability to directly address the roots of your concerns, deploying targeted suggestions that speak directly to your subconscious, where the real change takes place.

Opting for a session that aligns with your personal aspirations or challenges is straightforward, yet the potential benefits are profound. As you engage with a download that mirrors your needs, you are likely to notice a more pronounced responsiveness within yourself. This is because the therapy is speaking the language of your subconscious, tapping into and recalibrating the deep-seated narratives that govern your behaviours and emotions.

It is also worth noting that the journey of personal development is not static but evolves over time. As you progress with one aspect of your life, new areas for growth may emerge. Dr Postlethwaite's diverse range of hypnotherapy downloads accommodate this evolutionary process, offering the flexibility to shift focus as your journey unfolds. You might begin with a download aimed at enhancing relaxation and find that, as your stress levels decrease, you are drawn to sessions that promote confidence or motivation.

What sets this approach apart is the recognition that you are the architect of your own healing journey. With Dr Postlethwaite's hypnotherapy downloads, you are afforded the autonomy to shape your path to wellness, selecting and switching between sessions as your needs and goals evolve. This dynamic interaction not only empowers you but also enhances the therapeutic experience, ensuring that the benefits of hypnotherapy are fully harnessed to support your individual trajectory towards a more fulfilled and balanced life.

Testimonials and Success Stories

The journey of self-improvement and mental health enhancement through Dr Postlethwaite's hypnotherapy downloads is illuminated by a plethora of testimonials and success stories. These narratives, rich in personal victory and transformation, offer a glimpse into the life-changing potential of expertly guided hypnotherapy. Individuals from various walks of life share how these downloads have catalysed profound changes in their outlook, habits, and overall well-being.

One such story comes from a person who struggled with chronic insomnia for years, finding little relief through conventional treatments. They recount how, sceptical at first, they decided to try one of Dr Postlethwaite's sessions focused on sleep improvement. The results were nothing short of miraculous for them, with improved sleep patterns emerging within just a few weeks, leading to enhanced energy levels and a more positive mood throughout their day.

Another compelling account is from an individual battling severe anxiety, which hampered their ability to engage in social situations and perform effectively at work. Through regular engagement with Dr Postlethwaite's anxiety-specific hypnotherapy downloads, they experienced a significant reduction in their anxiety symptoms. They describe feeling a newfound sense of calm and confidence, attributes that have fundamentally changed their approach to life's challenges and interactions with others.

Further testimonials touch on a range of issues, from overcoming deep-seated phobias to managing chronic pain and quitting smoking. Each story is unique, yet a common theme resonates throughout: the transformative power of accessing and reprogramming the subconscious mind under the guidance of Dr Postlethwaite's experienced hand. Individuals express gratitude not only for the symptomatic relief they've achieved but also for the deeper self-awareness and personal growth they've experienced as a direct outcome of their hypnotherapy journey.

These success stories are not just accounts of personal triumph; they serve as beacons of hope for others who may be considering hypnotherapy as a path to wellness. They underscore the efficacy and impact of Dr Postlethwaite's work, highlighting his ability to facilitate meaningful, lasting change through the power of hypnotherapy. As more people come forward to share their experiences, the narrative around hypnotherapy continues to evolve, further establishing its validity and versatility as a tool for personal transformation.

Addressing Common Concerns and Misconceptions

Venturing into the realm of hypnotherapy, it's understandable that one may harbour certain reservations or misunderstandings, particularly with the myriad of myths surrounding the practice. Dr Postlethwaite's hypnotherapy downloads aim to demystify the process, ensuring that you can embark on this journey with confidence and a clear mind.

One prevalent concern is the fear of loss of control during hypnosis. It's a common misconception that being under hypnosis might compel one to act against their will or reveal personal secrets. However, this couldn't be further from the truth. Hypnotherapy places you in a state of heightened awareness and focus, where you remain fully in control and conscious of your surroundings. The essence of these sessions is to empower, not override, your autonomy and decision-making abilities.

Another area of uncertainty often lies in the effectiveness of hypnotherapy, especially when delivered through downloads at home. Some may wonder if these recordings can match the efficacy of in-person sessions. It's essential to understand that the potency of hypnotherapy stems from the quality of the therapeutic guidance and your receptiveness to the process. Dr Postlethwaite's extensive experience and nuanced understanding of the therapeutic process are encapsulated within each download. This ensures that, regardless of the medium, the therapeutic integrity and potential for impactful change remain intact.

There's also a narrative that hypnotherapy is a 'quick fix' for deep-seated issues, leading to unrealistic expectations about the speed of results. While hypnotherapy can produce remarkable outcomes, it is crucial to approach it with a mindset geared towards gradual and sustainable improvement. The journey to personal growth and healing is a process, one that may require time and repeated sessions to achieve the desired transformation. Patience and persistence, coupled with the high-quality guidance provided by Dr Postlethwaite's downloads, pave the way for genuine, long-lasting change.

Finally, the bespoke nature of Dr Postlethwaite's hypnotherapy downloads address any concerns that a one-size-fits-all approach might not suit everyone's unique needs. Each session is designed with the flexibility to cater to a wide array of issues, ensuring that your individual journey towards wellness is supported in the most relevant and effective way possible.

By engaging with these sessions, you're not merely undergoing a passive experience; you're actively participating in a scientifically backed process designed to foster self-discovery, healing, and empowerment. With Dr Postlethwaite's expertise guiding you through each step, hypnotherapy can be a transformative tool in your pursuit of well-being, free from the common misconceptions that may have once stood in your way.

Chapter 5

How to download your session

1) I will be sending you a text to your mobile phone; the text will look something like this:

https://www.dropbox.com/scl/fi/jeh0inlfjj1chal5kx7 f6/sample oflink.mp3?rlkey=q2xy2Hwghum9yf2u9iyu5c37

(please note the above is not a live link, it is only an example)

2) When you click on the text you phone will open, please look to the very bottom of the screen where you will see two buttons: (fig1)

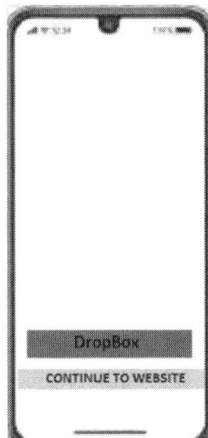 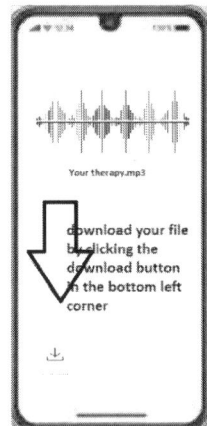

(Fig1)   (Fig2)

Unless you are a Dropbox subscriber already do not press the blue Dropbox button, instead press the grey button which is labelled Continue to website.

3) At this point you will see your therapy on the screen along with a play button (Fig 2). I would not recommend playing it at this stage as the quality could be affected by your download speed. If you look in the bottom left-hand corner of your screen you will see a download Icon, click on this and follow the onscreen instructions.

4) The file will begin to download, once download has completed which should not normally take more than about 20 seconds you will be asked if you want to save the file, click YES.

5) The file is now saved on your phone until you choose to delete it.

How to safely and effectively use your session.

a) Find a place where you can be comfortable, and you would be safe if you fell asleep. **Under no circumstances should you use your recording whilst driving or operating machinery**.

b) Begin to play your recording and follow the verbal instructions that I give you.

c) If you are using the recording at bedtime and you want to go to sleep then before commencing the play think to yourself 'I will ignore the wake-up instruction' this may take a few times to practice, but soon you will play the recording and not wake up until morning, having had a wonderful restful sleep.

d) Listen to your recording at least once a day for at least one month. If you are having a bad day you can use it more than once, and if you want to continue past the month then you can, you cannot overdose with relaxation.

e) Just enjoy and allow the changes to happen for you.

Printed in Great Britain
by Amazon

57513906R00031